The Little things they do not tell you about Iguinal Hernia Surgery and Recovery

I0436545

Written by Glenn D. Andrews

This is lifestyle advice, for medical advice please see you physician.

Hernia surgery and recovery

In late October 2013, I finally received the official diagnoses of the pain that I had not told my wife about! From July 2013 until my diagnoses I could not figure out what I did or did not do to cause this throbbing pain and lump that would go away when I lay down. Even crazier when I pushed on the lump in my groin the area would flatten out and it would appear normal, except for the pain. The Internet is a beautiful tool because a little research goes a long way. However, there is nothing that compares to an official diagnoses that comes from a Doctor. As I thought and was confirmed by my physician and subsequent surgeon I had an inguinal hernia. I literally was putting off going to the Doctor, until one day I sneezed and I thought my guts were going to come out! Finally, I told my wife and appointments were scheduled and I saw both doctors within three days.

Oh arrogant, cocky me! I was lifting weights, riding my bike 40 miles a week and running like I was in my twenties. When this all took place I had just turned 50 years old and felt great. The surgeon who was in his thirties indicated he needed to get into the physical condition I was in. So, I had what is called the open hernia repair surgery which was recommended because of my lifestyle (weightlifting, cross training and strength conditioning). This was the best option for me and you must consult with your surgeon what will be best for you and your lifestyle. So, I did the research between the open surgery and Laparoscopic and the open hernia surgery would minimize me getting another hernia. My ego and macho on a scale of 1- 10 was a Big Ten. I was 200 lbs. and 6 feet of fifty-year-old stud!

I never had any kind of surgery other than dental surgery and I was confident that I would handle hernia surgery like a champ.

My home indoor gym!

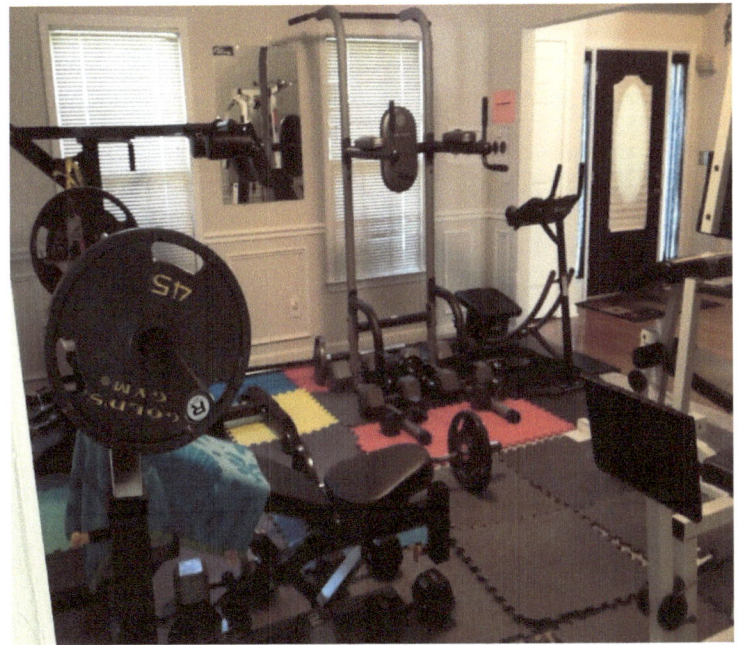

The outdoor oasis! Pull up, dip and push up bars.

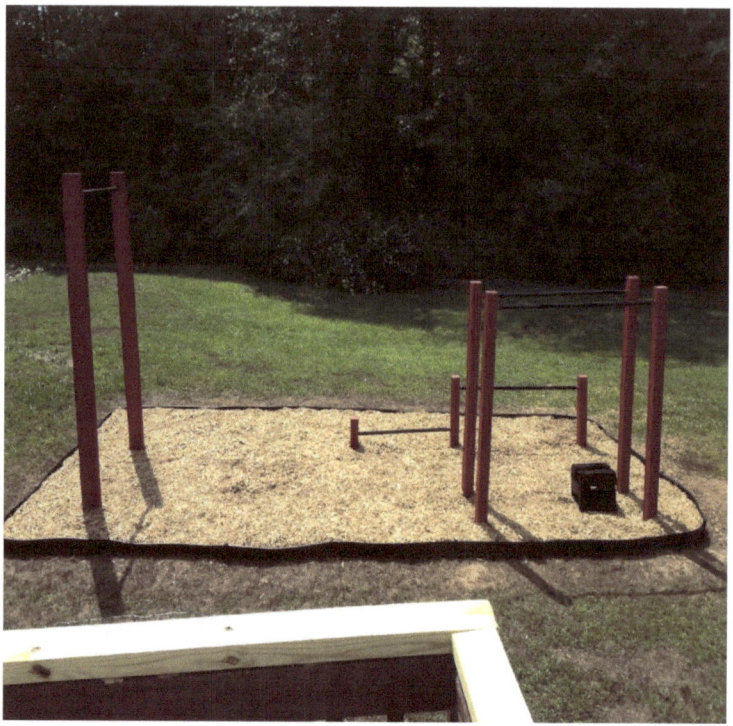

Hopefully, these pictures give you an idea about my

fitness life and how being diagnosed and having

hernia surgery affected my life and the adjustments

and changes you have to make.

Hernia surgery and recovery

The hernia pre-op and post-op information you receive from your surgeon or doctor will be thorough. Ask questions? Ask questions? Do not be scared to ask questions.

The information goes over the process from the day before the surgery until you come back a week to three weeks later for a follow-up after the surgery. However, there are several things you can do to minimize the discomfort that you are going to go through.

So, these are the top things you can do to be better be prepared for hernia surgery.

1. Depending on the amount of time you have before your scheduled surgery eat some of the foods you enjoy, but try to eat as "clean" or as healthy as possible. Eating healthy will play a major role in your recovery because during this time going to the bathroom will be physically challenging and the pain pills will disrupt your bowel movement. Additionally, your metabolism may slow down after the surgery and if you are eating healthy your body weight will adjust slowly. My body weight went from 200 lbs. to 192 lbs., and now I am 206 lbs. and my body is still adjusting ten months later. The foods I stocked up on to take the pain pills were Jell-O, Fruit cups, crackers, and peanut

butter. For fluids water, Gatorade and Pedia-lyte! Yes Pedia-lyte to keep you from becoming dehydrated. As much as you will not want to move! You will have to eat something so you can take your pain pills and this leads to # 2.

2. Prior to the surgery I was giving a pulmonary breathing test and watch a short video on the execution and purpose of the test. Boy, I thought this was a strange test to take just before surgery! But, again we are talking about the core of your body and the ability to breathe and or breathe deeply may be stressed. Additionally, I was so happy and thankful I did not have a cold or was dealing with seasonal allergies! Sneezing would have been the worst thing ever.

When you leave the hospital, hopefully you will be riding in a car. Preferably, a cushy, luxury sedan. First, you will be wheeled to the car so you can be driven home and the first test will be to get out of the wheelchair and into the car! A SUV or Truck may be too high to get into unless you are feeling real Spartan! Go for it. This has been the best advice from friends who have gone through this surgery, because the ride home will be memorable. You will feel every bump in the road and every time you come to a stop! It may be one of the longest rides you ever take that you cannot wait to end. Depending, on the area of your surgery be aware of how the seatbelts cross your body. Once you arrive at home, you will need assistance getting out of the car, so walking is not a problem lifting your legs for steps and stairs will be a challenge. This is where friends and family really will be needed. The scar for your open hernia surgery is in your groin area so you will be advised on the type of clothes to wear the day of the surgery. If you are shy! You will need a significant other, wife or husband to help you change clothes. I did not take a shower for a few days after surgery! But, I was not expending any energy or sweating! By the third day you should be able to change clothes and brush teeth! I know it sounds crazy, but it will all make sense.

3. You will be prescribed pain pills, serious pain pills –Take them .Coordinate the scheduling of your dosage of pain pills so you can sleep at night. I tried to take my last

pain pill of the day between 9 pm and 12 am, so at the very least you are not up at night due to pain. Everyone has a different pain tolerance, and if you are anything like me and I do not enjoy taking pills for anything. But, in this case you have to put that thought process aside so your body can heal. The hernia surgery is in the core of your body, and you do not realize how much you utilize your core to get out of bed, rise from a chair or reach for a phone or T.V. remote. So, whatever the duration and prescription you are giving to you by your doctor, follow the instructions.

4. Get all your linen cleaned prior to surgery! For the first few days you will not be able to take a shower do to pain and based on the type of bandages over your surgery area.

My doctor had a body glue and bandage over my surgery area which was nice. From the 2nd to 3rd week I could remove the glue with finger nail polish remover. Yes, finger nail polish remover but I discovered finger nail polish remover is cold! So, if you have the glue for bandage, when you take a shower have an extra face towel to be utilize with the finger nail polish remover to soak the surgery area. I ran the water as hot as I could stand it into the face towel, removed the water and poured the finger nail polish remover into the towel. Then just soak that area to remove the glue. This was process I did over a week and half removing small sections over time. If you do not start this process, once the hair begins to grow in that region you will be facing pain in area that is already sensitive.

5. Although the Lazy boy, sofa and bed can be comfortable for a while, hopefully you are beginning to get uncomfortable and this means it is time to start walking and getting the strength back. This is critical for getting your strength, metabolism and system moving. Most importantly if you have not had a BM (bowel movement), once you are up walking with minimal challenges you will make it to the bathroom. I used a cane, the door; the wall and a chair to get around and lean on in the house to walk back and fourth down the hall. The one thing I did not do for about a week and a half was walk up and downstairs. If you have bedroom upstairs you will be stationed there for a

while. What some friends with upstairs bedrooms have done was to set up in a downstairs guest bedroom and not go upstairs until the strength was back. Just keep in mind proximity of where you will sleep and the bath room has to be the shortest distance! You may not have a BM, but you will have to urinate because of the fluid intake when you take your pain pills.

6. I will tell you, 10 feet to the bathroom will be the incredible journey that will seem like an eternity. This is where your mind, body and faith have to get on the same page. As much as you do not want to get up, you have to start moving so you can get your system going, you have to take pain pills with food, which you have to ingest along with fluids but it is painful moving! But you have no

bowel movement! But you have to go to the bathroom on false alarms! This is what they call the irony of the hernia surgery, again even at these stages recovery if something is out of the ordinary do not hesitate to call your Doctor.

7. Hopefully, within a week you are up and walking, your system is functioning and you are able to eat at the table! Then you should have had your first shower, and for men (and women) a chance to shave and just get clean. To brush your teeth, take a shower, shave and be clean while putting on clothes is a milestone. This may be also an opportunity to go outside and even take a drive. Now, must of this depend on the degree of your pain and your recovery? Keep in mind you cannot take pain medicine

and drive, this is a Big NO! NO! I did not drive until about two weeks from the day of the surgery, but I went to a close friend's funeral a week after my surgery. My wife drove; I wore suspenders, and had a cane. I was on pain medication to be able to handle the drive and be as comfortable as possible during this time.

8. As I stated earlier I have a fitness lifestyle, but my occupation during this time involved heavy lifting and twisting. There are universal recovery times and physical limitations spelled out by your doctor, health insurance and your employer. They called it light duty for my occupation, which involved minimal lifting of anything beyond 45 lbs. As you get going and go back to work you have to define the line between

discomfort and pain. I will also say the line between discomfort and pain has to be defined at home. I started slowly working out strictly on machines and walking on the treadmill before I was scheduled back to work. There were two exercises I did not do it all, and to this day I only do about 20-30 repetitions. I no longer do roman chair ab exercises because my form has me stretching between my upper thigh and abdominal area. I gave my roman chair to friend training to become a police officer.

The other exercise or equipment was the ab

wheel.

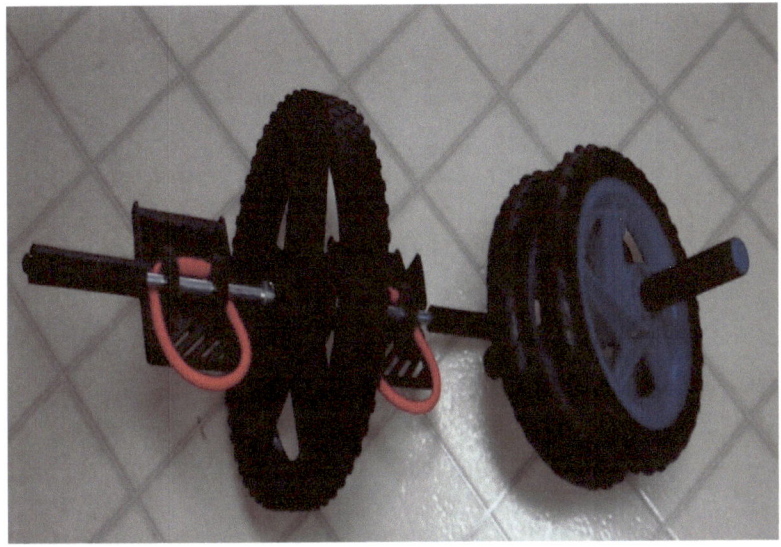

This is the cheapest and best abdominal

equipment on the planet.

 If you improve your diet, up your cardio

and exercise with the ab wheel, you will get

a tighter midsection. As much as I love my

ab wheel I had to stop doing them until I had

overall strength to be stabilized. I knew

how I could physically work so I had the

19

doctor be more clear, precise and specific about limitations and gave that information to my human resources department. So, be honest about where you are in your recovery and communicate that to your doctor, employer and your health insurer.

9. As you recover and gain limited strength and mobility you must adhere to the weight lifting limitations. If you are not allowed to lift anything weighing more than thirty pounds do not do it! You will not be putting everything on scale to see if it meets the weight requirement, however you must use your common sense and allow your friends and family to move or lift items for you. This stage in your recovery will be the most difficult to deal with, especially if you are a macho he-man that lifts trucks, trees and

mountains. When the wife comes in with groceries you may be tempted to do the normal 2 to3 grocery bag grab, don't do it! This is what teenagers are for, put them to work! If your hernia injury was anything like mines, I do not know the specific day, time, movement or what I did… But I plan on not do whatever it was not again.

10. Weight gain/loss and metabolism now becomes the small hurdle that can be mastered with patience and planning. The combination of exercise and nutrition during the recovery time is crucial in getting back to your physical performance especially if you were very active prior to your surgery. I started walking with the intent to getting back to running. I have a walk program on my treadmill that varied the speed of

walking between 3.0 and 4.0 mph. At this speed it took about 20 minutes to walk a treadmill mile. The goal was to increase the speed of walking until was safe to jog and in increments get my time down to a 7 minute jogging mile. My recovery was during the winter so the majority of my aerobic activity was spent between my spin bike and treadmill. Depending on your comfort or discomfort bicycles may not be for you. However, I found that my spin bike was not that uncomfortable along as I did not get into a fitness ride similar to a spin bike class. The approach with riding exercise bikes is to progressively add tension to the wheel. My indoor bike riding was kept between 4-6 miles, 2 to 3 times a week. There were some days I did "two a day" workouts and this was about three months after my surgery. For those who are serious cyclists there riding regimen would have a lot more miles and intensity. A cyclist's goal would be to get back to high performance cycling, whereas this premise is geared towards stabilizing weight gain and getting back to some normalcy. This also can be applied to those of you who are serious runners. A runners schedule is intense, I know because my wife and son run marathons and cross country races. For both the serious cyclist and runners your recover depends on your comfort level and intensity. But, patience and safety is the key.

11. Not being able to work out and lift weights was very difficult due to the fact it was the other piece of the puzzle in stabilize my

metabolism and weight. I was not to lift anything over 40 lbs. for 3 months based on how well my recovery was going and my follow up surgeon visit. Everyone is unique and the human body does not follow a calendar! The time periods for the stages of recovery vary from person to person. I had read story about a pro football player that had hernia surgery and was back at practice and in full contact in three weeks! All I can say is either he was special, or he had some special medicine…. I am just saying. In my opinion my recovery and strength went well because as difficult as it was I stayed away from heavy lifting and free weights. Workout machines are the best way to build your strength, stamina and assist you in getting back to lifting with free weights.

Workout machines stabilize and balance weight. Now I prefer free weights over machines, however these are the kind of adjustment mentally you have to make to get back healthy. Furthermore, if you are a serious weightlifter, bodybuilder and really into heavy weightlifting you have to find those exercises that physically and mentally work for you. I do not know if it is good or bad to not think every time you working out intensely you might get a another hernia? I do believe you improved your technique, form and concentration. You have to approach you fitness regimen with clarity, listen to your body and follow your doctor's instructions.

This machine was my therapy:

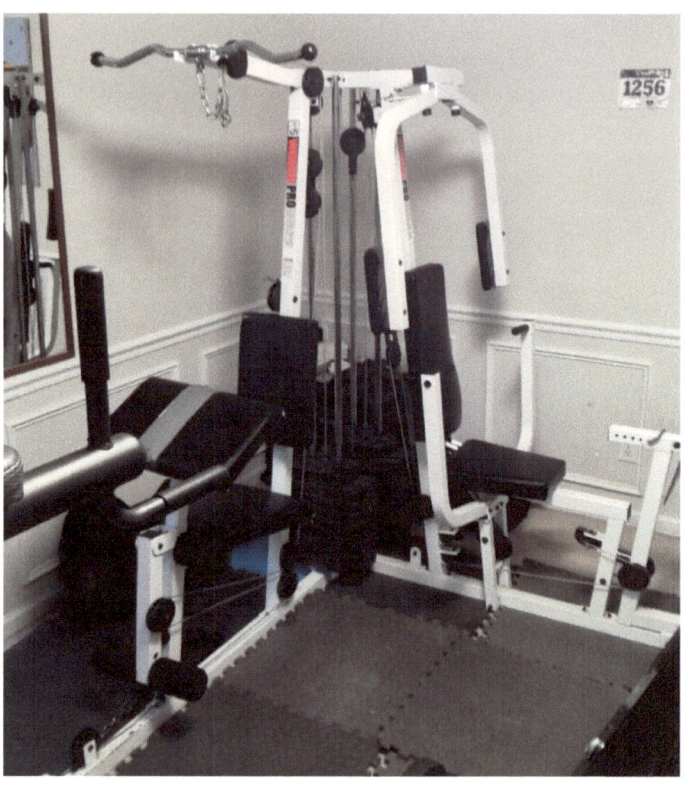

12. The old saying goes "losing weight and
body fat happens at the table, not at the
gym". If you are lucky and your metabolism
and weight stabilizes as you fully recover

you are the lucky one. I had to take into

consideration my body type which is an

endomorph.

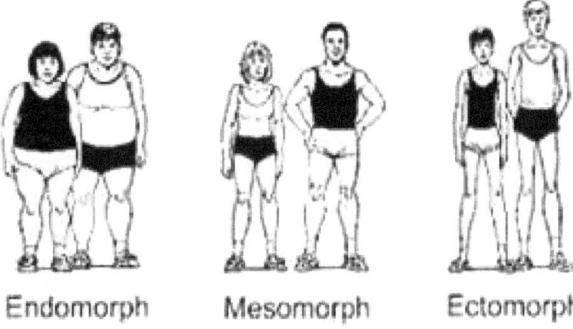

Endomorph   Mesomorph   Ectomorph

Courtesy of http://creativehealthyliving.com

13. About two years ago I was doing research

on vegetarian and vegan diets and I

discovered green smoothies. The next

discovery was how to blend and make

smoothies without the blender mess!

On father's day my wife and kids bought me

a Vitamix blender and it is the best gadget!!

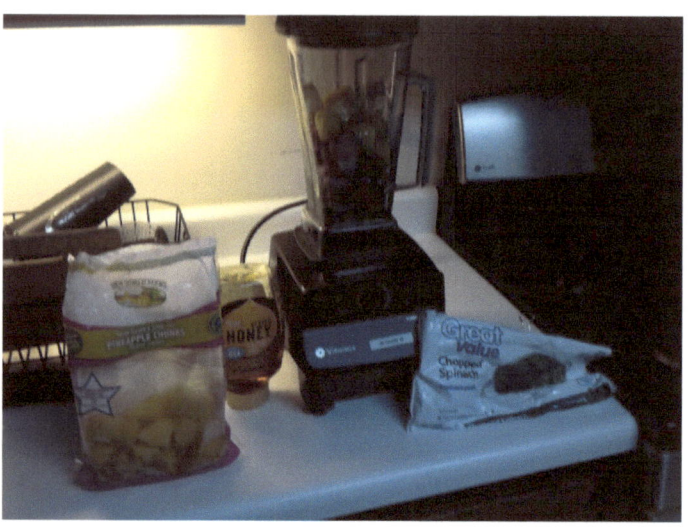

Prior to surgery I was already supplementing

my diet with green smoothies made with

different fruits mixed with broccoli, kale or

spinach. Monday through Friday I would

have a slice of turkey, a cup of fruit and a 20

oz. of protein drink made 1% milk, water

and protein or drink a green smoothie.

Although, my nutrition was the same as

28

before the hernia surgery my weight went from 200 lbs. to192 lbs., and then up to 215 lbs. and my clothes were fitting tight within 3 months! I easily could have gone up to 220 lbs. and beyond. My diet was 80 % healthy foods and 20% whatever I wanted, and this included KFC, I-hop pancakes and Papa John's pizza. The rapid weight gain, slow metabolism forced me to make some nutritional adjustments that included green smoothies for breakfast and lunch and yogurt as a snack.

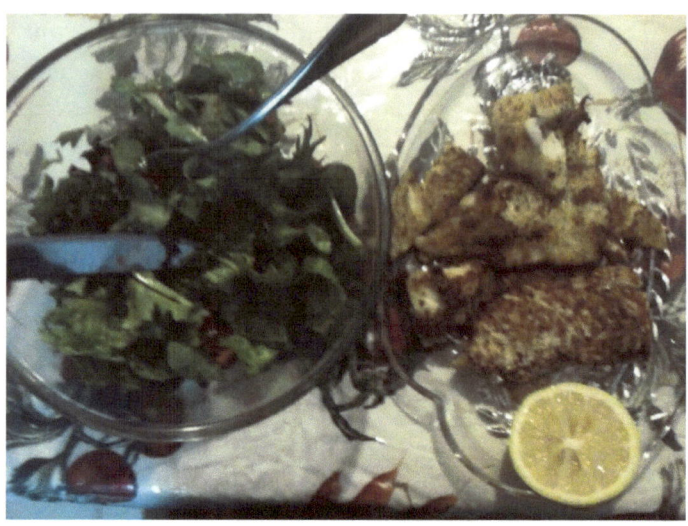

For dinner I would have a salad with fish, chicken breast or steak. There has been a lot of discussion about gluten, breads and starches and removing them completely from your diet. But, for this you have to make your own judgments. I cut back on my rice and bread intake. I also cut back on my portions and eating after 8:p.m.

I do eat limited amounts of starches and bread. Also by eating time, I mean you should try to cut back on eating heavy meals of any kind just before you went to bed.

Additionally, I tried eating food groups

within a window of being utilized. For

example for brunch I would have baked

lemon pepper chicken wings with apple. I

know it sounds crazy but it worked!

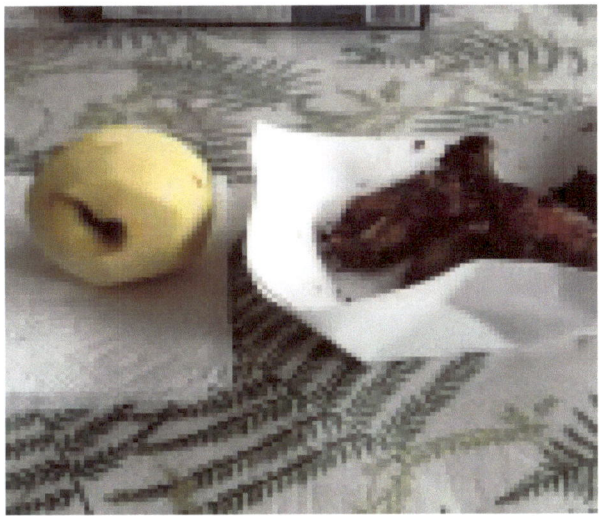

I am not a soda, Gatorade or PowerAde

drinker! You have to drink water and lots of

it. Being transparent I ran into a problem of

not having enough energy and I began to

31

drink coffee in the afternoon for energy. As my strength came back, weight came down and metabolism stabilize I no longer needed coffee or any type of energy drink. The key is keeping the energy up and maintaining a positive attitude. For some recovering from hernia surgery is easy, and others had major difficulties. There are many factors that influence how your body normalizes from hernia surgery including age, sex, level of physical activity and lifestyle.

If you were not eating healthy before your hernia surgery you need to start and if you were eating healthy prior to surgery adjust your portions and the times you eat.

I delayed going to my doctor initially, once I went to my doctor/surgeon and had a diagnosis of an inguinal hernia I immediately scheduled my surgery. Do not delay seeing a doctor and asking as many questions as you can think of. This surgery is to your core and you have to prepare prior to the surgery and after the surgery. My ego had to take a backseat to the doctor's instruction and common sense. Serious athletes, novices and those who do not workout have to get moving as soon as possible and listen to your body. More than likely improper lifting form or even a sneezed could have caused the hernia. But, as you get back into your routine take your time, use good form and follow the weight limitations prescribed by your physician. As

33

you recover you may find that your weight and metabolism maybe out of sync. The key to jump starting your nutritional recovery is "eating clean" and being aware how your body utilizes what you eat. Finally, some more good advice I received from friends and family, was do not delay getting the surgery done. Although you will have some challenges the human body is remarkable and you will be glad you took care of your hernia sooner than later. Finally, this is not medical advice, this is lifestyle advice! Consult your physician as soon as possible if you think you may have a hernia or any other health condition.

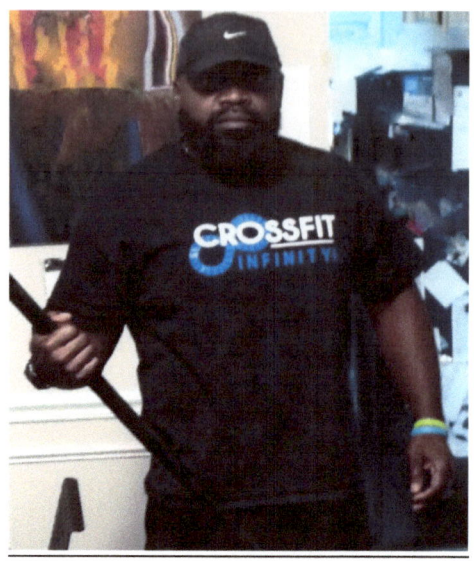

Glenn Darryl Andrews was born in Las Vegas, Nevada in 1963 and grew up in San Diego, California. An undergraduate of Morehouse College with a degree in Economics, M.B.A. from South University, Six Sigma Lean Green Belt from Emory University and a personal trainer. A social activist, mentor and fatherhood advocate was stunned to discover minimal information on the nuances of hernia surgery and recovery. So, these are the adjustments and processes Glenn implemented to heal and get back to his active lifestyle.